Edson Barbosa

Experimental chronic poisoning by Palicourea marcgravii in goats

Edson Barbosa

Experimental chronic poisoning by Palicourea marcgravii in goats

ScienciaScripts

Imprint

Cover image: www.ingimage.com

This book is a translation from the original published under ISBN 978-613-9-65331-7.

Publisher:
Sciencia Scripts
is a trademark of
Dodo Books Indian Ocean Ltd. and OmniScriptum S.R.L publishing group

120 High Road, East Finchley, London, N2 9ED, United Kingdom
Str. Armeneasca 28/1, office 1, Chisinau MD-2012, Republic of Moldova, Europe
Printed at: see last page
ISBN: 978-620-7-86669-4

Index

ACKNOWLEDGEMENTS

Firstly, I thank God for believing in me at times when I even doubted whether I would be able to complete the project. Thank you, eternal Father, for giving me the health, the peace I needed and all the resources to get this far.

To my beloved mother, Verônica de Figueiredo, for her example of effort, dedication and commitment. Not forgetting all the support she provided during the most difficult times throughout my journey.

My sisters and nephews, for bearing with me during the times when I was stressed and anxious. Thank you very much for the pleasant moments during the battle.

I would like to thank my grandmother Teca, who passed away during this stage of my life, on a necropsy day in the field. Unfortunately, she couldn't physically accompany our victory, but wherever she is, I'm sure she's cheering us on. Thank you so much for everything.

A special thank you to my animals, who always have a great time when I come home exhausted, teaching me that life is made up of good times.

I thank God for having put such a special person in my life, Fefa.

To Professor Márcio Botelho, for the opportunity and guidance throughout the work. Thank you very much.

Professor Luciana Sonne, for her example as a person and, above all, as an educator. To everyone at LPV-UnB, for their help, advice, personal and professional development. Thanks.

I would like to thank the great Augusto Moscardini, the couple Seu Nitin (the biggest weed collector) and Dona Ana. To my friends Rafael Gontijo, Saulo Pereira and Breno dos Santos, for the days of collecting in the middle of the forest, picking up ticks as a gift while we harvested the Palicoureas.

To my daily work mates during the 10 months at the CMO, Antonio, Zé, Gilson, Claudio, and all the trainees, especially Eduardo and Jânio. Thanks.

I'd like to thank Denise Salgado for her patience and help. Thank you very much for everything, my dear.

I thank you all because, in one way or another, you are part of who I am today in life. In some way you have helped me to improve as a person. Thank you.

To CAPES for the grant and to all the staff at the Sheep Management Centre at Unb's Água Limpa Farm for all their support in carrying out the project.

Thank you!

CHAPTER 1

Bibliographical review

1.1 The plant

Palicourea marcgravii is the most important plant causing sudden death in cattle farming in Brazil. Popularly known as "cafezinho", "erva-café", "vick", "erva de rato", it is a shrub from the Rubiaceae family, found almost everywhere in Brazil, with the exception of Mato Grosso do Sul and the Southern Region. It is considered by many authors to be one of the main toxic plants of interest to livestock in Brazil, due to its wide distribution, high toxicity, accumulative effect and good palatability. The presence of a small amount of the plant in the region is enough for cases of poisoning to occur. Even after desiccation, the leaves preserve their toxicity (Tokarnia & Dobereiner, 1986). In this way, cattle become intoxicated naturally, without the need to starve, as all they need is access to the woods and capoeiras (Tokarnia et al. 2012). Ingesting a small amount of leaves can cause sudden death, especially when the animal is stimulated. Despite being the most dangerous plant in Brazil, animal instinct does not protect cattle and buffalo from naturally ingesting the plant (Tokarnia et al. 2012).

Because of these characteristics, it causes severe economic losses throughout the country, except in the South, probably because of the subtropical climate. It is estimated that it is responsible for the death of more than 600,000 head/year of the national cattle herd (Nogueira et al. 2010). Others estimate that this figure could exceed one million animals per year. The occurrence of sudden death in cattle is directly linked to the presence of the plant on the property. In the Amazon region, where the highest number of animals die from poisoning caused by ingesting toxic plants, it is estimated that 80 per cent of losses are caused by ingesting P. marcgravii (Tokarnia et al. 2012).

These losses can be divided into direct - when they are caused by the deaths of intoxicated animals, falls in production and/or reproduction, or indirect - when they are necessary to prevent, with the use of herbicides, fences or other management measures adopted to prevent new outbreaks. In Brazil, the lack of reliable data on the frequency and death of animals caused by the ingestion of toxic plants makes it difficult to estimate the real losses (Riet-Correa & Medeiros 2001).

Due to the high toxicity of Palicourea marcgravii to livestock, the minimum doses required for intoxication of animals in the field are not yet fully known. The effects of chronic ingestion of small quantities of the plant can cause marked cardiotoxicity, characterised by marked heart failure (Tokarnia, Peixoto & Dobereiner, 1990; Tokarnia et al. 1986; Tokarnia et al. 1991).

Macroscopic and microscopic lesions are still rarely described in goats intoxicated by the plant, but it is suspected that they also occur (Tokarnia et al. 1991). P. marcgravii requires further studies to better understand its effects on animals and possible variations in clinical and pathological forms, with the aim of preventing intoxication through early and accurate diagnosis.

1.2 Active ingredient

Its active ingredient is monofluoroacetic acid or monofluoracetate - MFA. This substance is highly toxic, soluble in water, tasteless, odourless and colourless. Stable at over 110°C, it begins to decompose at 200°C and is extremely toxic to a large number of animal species. It was first produced in Belgium in 1896 (Chenoweth, 1949), but it was only in Germany in the 1930s that its toxicity was first observed (Alzert, 1971). In Poland, scientists studied the toxic effects of fluoracetate compounds, specifically fluoracetic acid, for more than 10 years (Chenoweth, 1949).

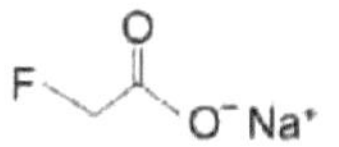

F O $O^- Na^+$

monofluoracetato de sódio.

Figure 01. Chemical formula of sodium monofluoracetate.

Years later it was detected in plants such as Dichapetalum spp. on the African continent

(Vickery and Vickery, 1972), Gastrolobium, Oxylobium, Acacia in Australia and Palicourea in South America. Australian plants contain up to 5 grams of the substance per kilogram of dried plants. In Brazil, it was identified by chromatographic technique (Oliveira, 1963, Lee et al. 2012) and later by high-performance liquid chromatography (HPLC) (0.20 to 0.24%). It was also identified using

from spectroscopy, at a concentration of 5.4gg/g of desiccated *Palicourea marcgravii* leaves, *and* 3.0pg/g in *Arrabidea bilabiata* (Krebs et al., 1994). A chromatographic peak similar to monofluoracetate was identified in *Mascgnania rigida* (Cunha et al. 2006). In plants of the *Dichapetalum* species, the concentration varies according to the part of the plant, with younger leaves containing a higher concentration of MFA than mature ones (Vickery and Vickery, 1972). However, in addition to monofluoracetate, other substances such as alkaloids, methyl salicylate, calcium oxalate crystals, tanoids, salicylic acid and 0-methoxybenzoic acid, caffeine, N-methyltyramine and 2-methyltetrahydro-P-carboline have been isolated from *P. marcgravii* (Peixoto et al. 2011).

1.3 Mechanism of action

The mode of action of MFA is based on the composition of fluorocitrate, its metabolite in active form. When it binds to acetyl-coenzyme A to form fluoroacetyl CoA, it replaces acetyl-coenzyme A in the Krebs cycle, reacting with citrate synthase, resulting in the synthesis of fluorocitrate, known as "lethal synthesis". (Colicho-Zuanaze & Satake, 2005). This compound blocks aconitase by competition, preventing the conversion of citrate into isocitrate, which results in its accumulation in the tissues, mainly the myocardium, liver and kidney. The high level of citrate binds to a large amount of calcium, causing marked hypocalcaemia, worsening arrhythmias and muscle tremors. As a result of the cycle being blocked, there is a marked decrease in the production of adenosine triphosphate (ATP) and, consequently, a drop in energy-dependent processes (Goncharov et al. 2006). This reduction in ATP production can reach 50%, caused by the blockage of oxidative metabolism, with a drop in acetate metabolisation and hepatic production of acetoacetate.

In addition to preventing the tricarboxylic acid cycle, monofluoracetate blocks the production of the neurotransmitter glutamate, a fact that is directly linked to the occurrence of seizures, since depletion of this neurotransmitter is one of the main causes (Colicho-Zuanaze & Satake, 2005).

When fluorinated compounds are metabolised by the liver, they can produce substances already known to have effects: narcotic analgesics - normeperidine derivatives, pesticides, antineoplastics, 5-fluoroacyl (Goncharov et al. 2006).

According to Kemmerling, 1996, the typical symptoms of "sudden death", however, are only observed in ruminants. This difference has yet to be explained. For the first time, two new molecules have been isolated from P. marcgravii that can act mutually by inhibiting the action of the enzyme monoamine oxidase A (MAO-A). Consequently, this inhibition would contribute to the stimulation of sympathetic receptors, which would further accentuate the toxic effects of MFA. In this way, the author considers that a small amount of MFA would be enough to cause sudden death in ruminants. On the other hand, it is believed that MFA is the main toxic principle responsible for most of the lesions caused by ingesting P. marcgravii, as it has recently been shown that the clinical picture in both experimentally intoxicated cattle (Nogueira et al. 2010) and sheep (Peixoto et al. 2011) is similar in several organs to those visualised in cases of intoxication by Brazilian plants that contain MFA in their composition, and therefore cause sudden death.

1.4 Metabolisation of monofluoracetate - MFA

The metabolisation of MFA, i.e. defluoridation, is carried out by anionic proteins with the action of glutathione-tranferase, but there are also cationic enzymes that are responsible for around 20% of the cytosolic defluoridation of fluoride. The main detoxification pathway is glutathione-dependent and occurs by nucleophilic attack on the carbon-beta atom, which results in the formation of a fluoride ion and S-carboxymethylglutathione, which is subsequently conjugated to proteins and excreted in the urine. In this way, the increase in fluoride ions in the bloodstream can be measured, making it useful in diagnosing MFA intoxication. The organs with the greatest defluoridation activity are, in descending order: liver, kidney, lung, heart and testicles. Its half-life and elimination from the body generally takes no less than two days, which is considered a potential risk of secondary poisoning (Goncharov et al. 2006). To date, no defluoridation activity has been found in the brain (Soifer and Kostyniak, 1983).

In cases of experimental intoxication, after oral administration of sodium MFA to sheep and goats at a dose of 0.1mg/kg body weight, the verified half-life of the substance was 10.8 hours and 5.4 hours, respectively. The highest concentrations of the toxin were seen 2.5 hours after oral administration, equivalent to 0.098p.g/ml in blood plasma, followed by kidney (0.057p.g/ml), (0.042p.g/ml) and liver 0.021 p.g/ml. After 96 hours, traces of the substance (0.008p.g/ml) were still detected in all tissues (Eason et al. 1994). In rabbits, the concentration of fluoracetate in the muscles, kidneys and liver was much higher than in the blood plasma (Goonerante et al. 1995).

1.5 Clinical signs of acute intoxication

The standard clinical signs of MFA intoxication are variable because they depend on the characteristic mode of administration (oral), the latency period, which varies from 0.5 to 6.0 hours, and variations in species-specific clinical signs. The length of the latency period depends on the time needed for the hydrolysis of fluoracetate into monoflouracetic acid to occur, as well as the production of a sufficient quantity of fluorocitrate, which will trigger the intracellular processes of a drop in energy production and thus manifest the clinical signs of intoxication. In the acute form, cardiac and nervous signs predominate, which can vary according to the species affected (Chenoweth, 1949).

These visible clinical signs apparently manifest themselves in three cycles. The first cycle is one of depression and apathy, lasting between 30 and 120 minutes. The second is one of excitement, lasting up to 30 minutes. Finally, the third, with signs of convulsions, lasts around 2 to 4 minutes. Death results primarily from asphyxiation during convulsions, as well as cardiac arrest or ventricular fibrillation and depression of the central nervous system, associated with cardiovascular and respiratory disorders (Chenoweth, 1949).

Susceptibility to toxic plants among animals varies widely as it depends on several variables such as: species, age, sex, individual resistance, acquired resistance, whether this is realised by selection or induced by different techniques that are used in the treatment and/or prophylaxis of certain types of poisoning (Pessoa, Medeiros & Riet-Correa, 2013). Sensitivity to MFA can vary greatly and can be attributed to differences in the degree of permeability of cell membranes and morphological differences. Functional differences between species can contribute to sensitivity to the substance (Buffa et al. 1977).

In order to adopt preventive measures, it is necessary to correctly diagnose poisoning by plants that cause sudden death (Barbosa et al. 2007).

1.6 Diagnosis of poisoning by MFA-containing plants

This diagnosis is based on obtaining as much information as possible about the history of deaths that have occurred on the property, as well as clinical signs of heart failure associated or not with exercise, checking the pastures for the suspect plant, correctly identifying the species of the toxic plant and then analysing it to detect and quantify the toxic substance causing the outbreak (Riet-Correa, & Medeiros, 2001).

The definitive diagnosis of sodium monofluoracetate intoxication in animals requires the detection of the substance using high-performance liquid chromatography (HPLC). This technique has proved suitable for quantifying MFA in plant samples, rumen contents and liver samples. However, in biological samples kept at room temperature, the identification capacity of the technique fell by around 50 per cent. The study suggested that biological samples should be analysed at a maximum of one week if they are not refrigerated (Minnaar et al. 2000).

Evaluating samples of plant leaves, tissues and blood taken during necropsy, i.e. post-mortem, using the same technique, proved to be effective in quantitatively determining the substance in samples of plants, liver and rumen content from intoxicated cattle (Cunha et al. 2006).

The prognosis for P. marcagravii poisoning is unfavourable, as depending on the amount of leaves ingested, it can cause sudden death in cattle (Tokarnia et al. 2012).

1.7 Experimental poisoning by MFA from plants containing it

In a study carried out on goats, doses of fresh P. marcgravii leaves ranging from 0.6g/kg to 1.0g/kg resulted in the death of more than two thirds of the animals. The time interval between the onset of clinical signs, stimulated by exercise, and the death of the animals ranged from one minute to two days, a longer interval than that observed in cattle and sheep. The main clinical signs seen were reluctance to move, walking with stiffened limbs, sternal decubitus with progression to abdominal and then lateral decubitus, muscle tremors, marked dyspnoea and death. Histopathology showed discrete foci of coagulation necrosis of cardiomyocytes, necrosis and vacuolisation of hepatocytes, while in the kidney, only one animal showed coagulation necrosis of the epithelial cells of the cortical urinary tubules (Tokarnia et al. 1991).

In South Africa, there have been reports of losses of ruminants with fibrotic changes in the myocardium, in animals that were kept in pastures where the plant D. cymosum (Gifblaar) was found. MFA has been detected in the composition of this plant, which is why, when ingested in large quantities, it can cause sudden death. However, if consumed in small quantities over a certain period of time, it can cause marked cardiac alterations. For this reason, a study of MFA intoxication in sheep was carried out in order to experimentally reproduce the typical lesions observed in sudden and chronic death caused naturally by the D cymosum plant on the continent (Shultz et al. 1982).

The toxin was administered to 17 Merino sheep at doses of between 0.05 -1.0 mg/kg/day. Microscopy showed that all the animals died acutely at a high dose or from prolonged exposure at a lower dose. Histopathological lesions in the heart muscle. The lesions were distributed along the atrial and ventricular walls, most commonly affecting the endocardium. In the chronic subacute form of intoxication, the lesions ranged from early degeneration to necrosis with no cellular response. In general, lesions in the myocardium were more common in acute cases. Prominent alterations were found mainly in the endocardium, such as the presence of numerous fibres that were swollen, swollen and stained less intensely with HE. In some cases there was a loss of striations and a rarefied cytoplasm, particularly in the perinuclear region.

Many of the areas of necrosis found were infiltrated mainly by lymphocytes and macrophages and some neutrophils. Fibroplasia and/or proliferation of sarcolemmal nuclei, sometimes accompanied by hypertrophy of myocardial fibres, was evident in some of the foci that were in the process of resolving. A discrete infiltrate of lymphocytes was observed in the interstitial connective tissues, scattered around the blood vessels in the myocardium. Although Purkinje fibres were not primarily involved, some fibres were surrounded by lymphocytes, fibroplasia, delimited by a focal myocardial lesion. In the other organs, apart from the congestion of most tissues, pulmonary oedema and slight nephrosis were observed in some animals; no noteworthy lesions were observed in the brain, liver, spleen, lymph nodes, suprarenal glands or skeletal muscles. Most of the sheep subacutely and chronically intoxicated with MFA did not die of acute heart failure and were euthanised. Apart from the pale, cooked-looking myocardium, no other noteworthy macroscopic lesions were visualised in the sheep's hearts. Although myocardial fibrosis in gousiekte (the African name given to rubiaceae intoxication in sheep and cattle) appears to be focal, it can be more diffuse and extensive, mainly restricted to the endocardial apex, interventricular septum and left ventricle. The lesions of MFA intoxication tend to be multifocal in nature, less generalised and evenly distributed in the myocardium (Shultz et al. 1982).

The authors conclude that there is little chance of reproducing the typical lesions of gousiekte (sudden death of ruminants due to ingestion of rubiaceae - Pachystigma pygmaeum) by administering MFA alone. Future attempts to experimentally reproduce these lesions should therefore be related to the dosage of the toxin in the plant (Shultz et al. 1982).

In the north-east, there is a shrub from the Rubiaceae family, P. aeneosfusca, which causes major losses due to sudden death in ruminants under natural conditions, especially when the animals are stimulated to exercise. Like P. marcgravii, its main active ingredient is monofluoracetic acid. This plant has lethal toxicity for goats at a dose of 0.65g/kg of fresh leaves, as well as showing a cumulative effect in consecutive daily administrations of 1/5 1/10 of the lethal dose. The main clinical signs observed in the intoxication of this plant from the northeastern region of Brazil were tachycardia, tachypnoea, falls, which progressed to death around 12 to 15 hours after oral administration. No noteworthy alterations were observed during the post-mortem inspection. Histopathology showed only hepatocyte degeneration (Passos, 1983). However, in the experimental intoxication of cattle by P. aeneofusca, the necropsy findings were negative. Histopathology showed marked hydropic-vacuolar degeneration associated with nuclear pyknosis of the epithelial cells of the distal convoluted urinary tubules in three cattle, and vacuolisation of hepatocytes in two of the three intoxicated animals that ingested single doses of fresh leaves (Tokarnia et al. 1983).

Studies with cattle were divided into two parts, the first using 30 animals, of which 28 died, the lowest lethal dose was 0.4g/kg of fresh P. marcgravii leaves, and the lowest that did not cause death was 0.5 g/kg. However, doses starting at 0.6 g/kg already produced serious clinical signs and the death of the animals. The second part used 11 cattle, 4 died, desiccated leaves were administered, the lowest dose that led to death was 0.29g/kg, and the highest that was not lethal was 2.0g/kg. In the experiment with repeated doses, 3 out of the 5 cattle died, always using desiccated leaves. The 3 animals received doses corresponding to 1/5 1/10/ 1/20 of the lethal dose, at 7-day intervals, for 25, 30 and 30 weeks respectively. As they didn't show any clinical signs, two of the cattle that had been receiving 1/5 1/10 weekly started receiving the doses daily. One of them died on the fourteenth daily administration of 1/5 of the lethal dose. Another bovine in the experiment, which received a total of 54 daily doses of 1/10th of the lethal dose, only showed mild signs for 48 hours when subjected to exercise. Most of the animals in the study died without being exercised, but the stimulus seems to have precipitated the appearance of clinical signs of intoxication (Tokarnia & Dobereiner, 1986).

In the experiment with fresh leaves, all 28 of the 30 animals assessed in the study fell ill. 14 animals were found dead and in the other 14, the clinical course varied from 1 to 10 minutes in 10 animals and from 19 to 85 minutes in the remaining four. The author only considered clear signs of intoxication. The clinical signs observed in the study with single doses of both fresh and desiccated leaves, both in those that died and those that recovered, in the order in which they appeared were: reluctance to move, more frequent urination, positive venous pulse, loss of balance, falling to the ground, muscle tremors, lateral decubitus, tachypnea, pedalling movements, opisthotonus, vocalisation, tonic convulsion and death. In the experiment with repeated doses that resulted in death, one of the animals showed dyspnoea, anorexia, apathy, sterno-abdominal decubitus, tachypnoea, positive jugular venous pulse, heart murmur, loss of balance, with a subsequent fall and death. In other cattle, anorexia, apathy, sterno-abdominal decubitus, difficulty moving, positive jugular venous pulse, slight muscle tremors were also observed, and they were later found dead. In 13 of the 28 animals intoxicated with single doses, there were no noteworthy necropsy findings. In the rest of the animals, the lesions found were discreet and consisted of pulmonary oedema and gallbladder insertion, pulmonary, hepatic, splenic and renal congestion, mucous membranes of the small intestine, mesenteric lymph nodes, epicardial haemorrhages and mucous membranes of the trachea (Tokarnia & Dobereiner, 1986).

In the experimental study, with the administration of single doses of fresh leaves of the plant, the main findings in the histopathological evaluation of the heart were intracellular oedema, characterised in the form of foci, in which there was vacuolisation of the cardiac fibres in 5 of the 28 cattle. Cardiomyocyte necrosis, characterised by marked eosinophilia of the cytoplasm, with loss of striations and nuclear pyknosis, was observed in 3 animals. According to the author, in addition to these alterations already described, areas of separation between the cardiac myofibres were seen in 9 cases, in which there were also focal areas with infiltrates of small round cells. In the liver, there was swelling of hepatocytes in 5 cases and vacuolisation of their cytoplasm in 13 animals. Necrosis in the form of cytoplasmic eosinophilia of hepatocytes, with condensed chromatin in only 1 case, and liver congestion in 4 cases. The kidney showed hydropic-vacuolar degeneration in 17 cases and albuminous-granular- vesicular degeneration in the cortex of the kidney in 3 cases (Tokarnia & Dobereiner, 1986).

Necropsy findings in cattle, sheep and goats with acute P. marcgravii intoxication are generally scarce or absent and consist of non-specific alterations such as cardiac hyperaemia, pulmonary and intestinal circulatory alterations. Histopathological changes in acute cases are also inconsistent and are characterised by hydropic degeneration of the epithelial cells of the distal renal convoluted tubules. In acute intoxication protocols, the cardiotoxicity of P. marcgravii has been characterised, and can be precipitated by exercise stimulation through hydropic degeneration of renal tubules and myocardial necrosis, inflammation and fibrosis (Tokarnia & Dobereiner, 1986; Tokarnia et al. 1990; Tokarnia et al. 1991).

In the northern region, there are reports that buffaloes die less from P. marcgravii intoxication, so these animals would be considered more resistant than cattle. However, apart from the fact that the resistance is actually greater than that of cattle, this can be explained by the preferential habitat of the respective species. Cattle inhabit both firm ground and flooded areas such as floodplains, where A. bilabiata grows, which, as well as being less toxic than P. marcgravii, is only consumed by cattle when they are hungry. Palicourea, on the other hand, is eaten by cattle on dry land even if they are not hungry, due to the plant's palatability. In this study, epidemiological data was collected that showed a lower number of deaths in buffaloes compared to cattle, even when both were on dry land. This proved that buffalo were at least six times more resistant than cattle to P. marcgravii poisoning. The author concluded that the lower number of buffalo deaths in the Amazon was not only due to this resistance to the toxic action of P.marcgravii, but for another reason, which would be the species' preferred habitat of the floodplain, which coincidentally is where A.bilabiata is found, which is less toxic than the former (Barbosa et al. 2003).

In a comparative toxicity study carried out in the northern region, assessing the sensitivity to P. juruana in buffaloes and cattle, it was suggested that the former would be about twice as resistant as cattle. In this experiment, the plant appeared to be more toxic than P. marcgravii, but the author did not know what to attribute the difference to (Oliveira et al. 2004).

Nogueira et al. 2010 suggested the need for further studies focusing on rumen microorganisms associated with the inactivation of sodium monofluoracetate.

1.8 Prophylaxis and experimental control

Experimental studies on the use of rumen detoxification techniques to prevent losses in ruminants intoxicated by plants that cause sudden death should be one of the main objectives of studies carried out in Brazil. Poison control techniques still lack the development of interdisciplinary research programmes that address the various aspects related to plants, especially the correct identification of the toxic substance responsible for deaths and economic losses (Riet-Correa, & Medeiros, 2001).

Greeg et al. (1998) produced genetically modified bacteria including a gene coding for the production of enzymes with dehalogenase activity, originating from one species of Moraxella sp, in another known as Butirivibrio fibrisolvins. After being inoculated into the rumen of a sheep, it proved promising in protecting against MFA intoxication. This enzyme is capable of hydrolysing the poison before it is absorbed. Recently in Brazil, a dehalogenase-producing microorganism was isolated and identified from the rumen of a goat, a fact that confirms that there is a possibility of adapting animals to consuming plants containing MFA because the bacterium would be present in the rumen contents even in animals that have never ingested these toxic plants (Camboim et al. 2012). Thus, it is suggested that by administering successive and increasing sub-doses of the plant, promoting adaptation of the microbiota, the population of these microorganisms capable of hydrolysing the poison could multiply and, consequently, protect the animals. This alternative has been proven, as the enzyme capable of hydrolysing the poison is more common among rumen bacteria than previously believed (Oliveira et al. 2013, Duarte et al. 2014).

In order to prevent outbreaks of Palicourea aeneosfusca intoxication, conditioned food aversion was developed in goats using small doses of desiccated P. aeneosfusca. After administering the daily dose of the plant, the animals ingested 175mg/kg body weight of lithium chloride via a rumen probe. In this study, it was found that it was possible to induce conditioned aversion to P. aeneosfusca for around 90 days by ingesting successive non-toxic doses of the plant (Oliveira et al. 2013).

An experimental study of intoxication by MFA and other Brazilian plants that cause sudden death was carried out on rats to evaluate the protective effect of acetamide. In this experiment, 9 of the 33 rats that were evaluated ingested P. marcgravii , one at a dose of 2.0g/kg and the other 4.0/kg , they received oral doses of acetamide one minute before the plant was administered. The one that received 2.0g/kg of leaves received 2.0g/kg of acetamide and the second 4.0g/kg respectively. The result suggests that acetamide has a satisfactory protective effect, being able to prevent the appearance of clinical signs and avoiding the death of the rats (Peixoto et al. 2011).

Subsequently, the author experimentally intoxicated cattle with sodium monofluoracetate and P. marcgravii in order to assess the protective effect of acetamide, administered just before ingesting both compounds. After a week, the cattle were re-intoxicated with the same compounds, but without the prior administration of acetamide and all the animals died, proving the protective effect of the component (Peixoto et al. 2012).Despite the protective effect against MFA, acetamide has negative effects on the body similar to those seen with glycerol monoacetate. Among the adverse effects are hyperglycaemia, metabolic acidosis, endothelial damage to capillaries and lysis of erythrocytes (Egyed & Schultz et al. 1986).

Table 00. Main plants causing sudden death in cattle in Brazil.

Family	**Scientific name**	**Popular name**	**Lethal dose**	**Incidence**	**Active ingredient**
Rubiaceae	Palicourea marcgravii	Rat weed, coffee.	0.6g/kg	North, North-East, Central-West, South-East	Monofluoacetic acid
Bignoniaceae	Arrabidea bilabiate	Lash, lash	2.5g/kg	North	Steroids Cardio-active
Malpighiaceae	Mascagnia pubflora	Corona	5g/kg	Centre-West, South East	Chromones

Source: Riet-Correa (2001).

As the clinical course of intoxication is usually super-acute, it is impossible to indicate any supportive therapy, as according to the literature, stimulating exercise can cause death. For this reason, it is recommended to avoid moving animals or herds as little as possible during the period when they are in pastures where P. marcgravii is found. This is because the plant has a cumulative effect, and its elimination is normally slow. According to observations made in the field by farmers and cowboys, it takes around five days for the toxin to be metabolised and excreted. However, in experiments carried out with single doses, a period of 48 hours was sufficient (Tokarnia et al. 2012).

It is recommended to fence off the areas where the plant is found, or pull it out by the roots, then apply herbicide to the area in an attempt to prevent further regrowth. This procedure has been used by farmers with satisfactory results (Tokarnia et al. 2012).

In the northern region, where around 80 per cent of sudden bovine deaths are attributed to P. marcgravii, it is better to breed buffaloes instead of cattle, as the former are more resistant (Barbosa et al. 2003).

CHAPTER 2

Clinicopathological investigation of experimental chronic intoxication of goats by Palicourea marcgravii.

Edson de F. G. Barbosa[1 2]

Palicourea marcgravii is considered to be the main toxic plant of interest to livestock in Brazil, but so far only the acute form of intoxication is well known. This study assessed the clinical and pathological changes in 10 goats chronically intoxicated by P. marcgravii. The animals were given 0.2 g/kg body weight of the fresh plant every day for 6 to 38 days. The goats' main clinical signs were anorexia, apathy, tachycardia, arrhythmia, positive jugular venous pulse and decubitus. At necropsy, the macroscopic findings were hydropericardium, pallor of the kidneys and myocardium, gelatinous atrophy of the cardiac fat, evidence of a hepatic lobular pattern and pulmonary oedema. The main microscopic findings were swelling and vacuolisation of cardiomyocytes, necrosis of cardiac fibres and a mononuclear inflammatory infiltrate in the myocardium. Diffuse hydropic-vacuolar degeneration was found in the kidneys. The findings showed a clinical-pathological picture in chronically intoxicated goats that was different from that observed in the acute form of P. marcgravii intoxication. These observations prove the risk to goats of ingesting the plant, even in small doses, resulting in the appearance of a clinical picture and serious lesions that are still little known and could be confused with other diseases.
INDEXING TERMS: Goat, Palicourea marcgravii, chronic intoxication, cardiotoxicity.

[1] Veterinary Hospital, University of Brasília (UnB), Via L4 Norte, Cx. Postal 4508, Brasília, DF 70910-970, Brazil.
*Author for correspondence: mbcastro(S)unb.br
[2] Sheep Management Centre - Água Limpa Farm - University of Brasília (UnB), Brasília, DF 71750-000, Brazil.
[3] Veterinary Hospital, Universidade Federal de Campina Grande, Patos, PB 58700-000, Brazil.

CHAPTER 3

INTRODUCTION

Palicourea marcgravii is considered the main toxic plant of interest to livestock in Brazil. Brazil, it is distributed throughout most of the country, with the exception of Mato Grosso do Sul and the Southern Region. In the Northeast, it has only been described in areas with good rainfall, and does not occur in the semi-arid or floodplains (Tokarnia et al. 2012). Its importance is reinforced by its wide distribution, good palatability, high toxicity and accumulative effect, being responsible for the death of 80 per cent of cattle poisoned by plants in the Amazon region (Tokarnia et al. 1986, Tokarnia et al. 1991, Tokarnia et al. 2012).

The fresh leaves of P. marcgravii contain monofluoroacetic acid (MFA), which causes sudden death in animals, even after ingestion of a single dose of 0.6 to 1.0 g/kg for cattle and goats respectively (Tokarnia & Dobereiner, 1986, Tokarnia et al. 1991).

In Brazil, most farm animals are raised extensively on native or cultivated pastures, as the main basis of their diet. For this reason, there is often greater access and exposure of animals to toxic plants, partly explaining the large number of losses in plant poisoning outbreaks recorded in Brazil (Pessoa, Medeiros & Riet-Correa, 2013).

In the Federal District (DF), the death of goats with neurological signs was observed, kept in areas with access to riparian forests, which contained small amounts of P. marcgravii and with signs of ingestion of the plant by the animals. At the time, a histological diagnosis of polyencephalomalacia was made. This lesion had previously been found in cattle suspected of being intoxicated by the plant (Ecco et al. 2004). These findings prompted a previous pilot study in goats with low and repeated doses (0.2g/kg body weight of fresh leaves of the toxic plant), where no alterations were detected in the CNS; however, severe degenerative-necrotic lesions appeared in the myocardium and the animals died.

To date, most studies on farm animals have aimed to determine the effect and toxic dose of P. marcgravii on the reproduction of acute intoxication, which is frequently observed in most outbreaks (Tokarnia, Peixoto & Dobereiner, 1986, Tokarnia, Peixoto & Dobereiner, 1990, Tokarnia et al. 1991, Barbosa et al. 2003).

The ingestion of small doses of P. marcgravii for prolonged periods, in areas with little availability of the plant, could also be involved in the death of animals, mainly due to severe heart damage, unlike the acute form of intoxication. It is also important to consider that small doses of plants containing MFA have been used to induce resistance in ruminants, in an attempt to prevent intoxication (Oliveira et al. 2013, Duarte et al. 2014), but could in some way cause heart damage to the animals.

The aim of this study was to investigate the evolution and clinical-pathological effects of chronic administration of fresh P. marcgravii leaves to goats.

CHAPTER 4

MATERIAL AND METHODS

The experiment was carried out at the University of Brasilia's Água Limpa Farm, in the Sheep Management Centre, from August to October 2013. Thirteen clinically healthy goats were used, seven of them of the Parda Alpina breed, 4 females and 3 males. The rest of the animals were all Saanem males aged between 6 and 8 months. The goats were kept in covered collective stalls with cement floors and wooden platforms, fed corn silage, commercial concentrate for goats, freshly chopped elephant grass (Pennisetum purpureum), commercial mineral salt for goats and fresh water ad libitum. Prior to the experiment, they were given monthly doses of anti-parasitic drugs (Closantel and Albendazole) during the period of food and environmental adaptation.

Ten goats (C1 to C10) received daily individual oral doses of 0.2 g/kg/animal of fresh P. marcgravii leaves. The plants were collected weekly from the forests of the Federal District and surrounding areas, on properties where there had previously been cases of intoxication in cattle. The plants were then stored in plastic bags refrigerated between 5 and 8 °C until they were administered to the animals. The control animals (C11 to C13) were kept under the same environmental and feeding conditions, but without ingesting the toxic plant.

In order to assess the evolution of chronic P. marcgravii intoxication as completely as possible, a daily clinical assessment was carried out in the morning, determining the duration and onset of clinical signs in the animals, with emphasis on assessing attitude (anorexia and apathy), heart rate and changes, respiratory rate, episcleral vessels and mucous membranes, jugular stasis and decubitus. The clinical examination was carried out up until the day before the animal was euthanised or died.

The animals that did not spontaneously die of intoxication were euthanised at 24 days and 39 days after starting to eat the plant. Two animals that resisted chronic intoxication for 38 days (C3 and C7) were then given a single dose of 2g/kg of fresh leaves of the plant, with the aim of determining whether they had developed resistance to the toxic principle (Oliveira et al. 2013). Goat C3 was challenged the day after the end of the initial experimental protocol and animal C7 after a 5-day interval. The control goats were euthanised at 39 days.

All the goats at the end of the protocol or those that were intoxicated, in agony or about to die were euthanised by barbiturate overdose (Concea, 2013). The animals were necropsied and organ fragments (heart, lungs, liver, kidneys, adrenal glands, spleen, central nervous system, intestines, pancreas, lymph nodes and skeletal striated muscle) were taken and fixed in 10% buffered formalin solution. The histological samples were routinely processed and histological sections were stained using the haematoxylin-eosin (HE) technique for evaluation under light microscopy.

CHAPTER 5

RESULTS

The main clinical alterations observed in goats chronically intoxicated by P. marcgravii are shown in **Table 1**. The onset of clinical signs occurred between 5 and 6 days after the start of the experiment, however, most of the animals showed alterations between 13 and 20 days. Most of the animals received the plant for at least 23 to 38 days, with the exception of two goats, which died prematurely at 6 and 16 days into the experiment. The minimum total dose of plant ingested/kg (DTI) that caused the death of one goat (C9) in just 6 days was 1.2g/kg. However, most of the animals received total doses of 4.6 to 7.6 g/kg until the end of the experiment.

Tachycardia (TAC), arrhythmia (ART), tachypnoea (TAP), engorged episcleral vessels (VEP) and sternal decubitus (DEC) were the main clinical signs observed in 100% of the chronically intoxicated goats. Apathy (APT), positive jugular pulse (PJP) were present in 90% of all the goats and anorexia (ANX) in 80%.

Goat C3, which was challenged with 2g/kg of the plant's fresh leaves 24 hours after the end of the experiment, showed similar clinical signs to the other animals, but 3 hours after the dose, it went into decubitus and remained apathetic until it died. Animal C7, when challenged with 2g/kg of fresh leaves of the plant 5 days after the last administration, showed no clinical signs for more than 12 hours, but was found dead 12 hours later.

The main necroscopic changes in the experimental animals were observed in the heart, kidney, liver, lungs and mucous membranes (**Table 2**). The most significant cardiac alterations were myocardial pallor (**Figure 1A**), hydropericardium (**Figure 1B**) and gelatinous fat atrophy. The kidneys of all the animals were pale (**Figure 1C**) and the liver showed a lobular pattern (**Figure 1D**) and diffuse congestion. The lungs of some animals showed mild to moderate oedema and congestion. The challenged animals (C3 and C7) showed macroscopic lesions similar to the other goats. The control animal showed no noteworthy macroscopic alterations.

Histopathological examination of the intoxicated goats showed alterations mainly in the heart. A summary of the most significant cardiac histopathological findings can be found in **Table 3**. The goats challenged (C3 and C7) with 2g\kg of fresh goat leaves showed histological lesions similar to the other goats.

Among the most significant cardiac lesions in the intoxicated animals, cardiomyocyte swelling and vacuolisation (**Figure 2A**) stood out due to their severity and multifocal to diffuse distribution. The cardiac fibres showed cytoplasmic expansion and vacuolisation, the latter characterised by a marked unstained perinuclear area.

The C3 and C7 animals, after being challenged with the plant, showed only tumefaction and discrete, focal vacuolisation of cardiomyocytes. The other tissues analysed showed similar histological lesions to the other goats.

Another important finding was individual necrosis of cardiomyocytes, with a sparse distribution and generally discreet intensity, characterised by cytoplasmic hypereosinophilia, loss of striations and sometimes caryopsia. Around the foci of necrosis, perivascularly and in the interstitium of the myocardium, there was a generally discrete mononuclear inflammatory infiltrate, made up predominantly of lymphocytes and macrophages (**Figure 2B**). In the left ventricle of only one of the goats (C5), discrete multifocal fibrosis was seen between the cardiomyocytes.

The interventricular septum, right and left ventricles were the most frequently affected regions and the main lesions were more intense. The right and left atria also showed the same alterations, but with less frequency and intensity.

Hydropic vacuolar degeneration of the renal tubular epithelium (**Figure 2D**) was present in all the intoxicated animals, ranging from mild to severe, with multifocal to diffuse distribution. On histopathological examination, the tubular epithelial cells showed translucent cytoplasmic vacuoles, karyopyknosis, karyorrhoea or absent nuclei.

The liver of only one of the goats (C9) showed moderate vacuolisation of hepatocytes in the central lobular region (**Figure 2C**). The hepatocytes had a slightly eosinophilic cytoplasm with a granular appearance, containing well-defined unstained vacuoles. Congestion and slight pulmonary oedema were found in the lungs of some of the goats in the experiment.

The only control animal (C11) that was euthanised showed no noteworthy microscopic changes in all the tissues analysed.

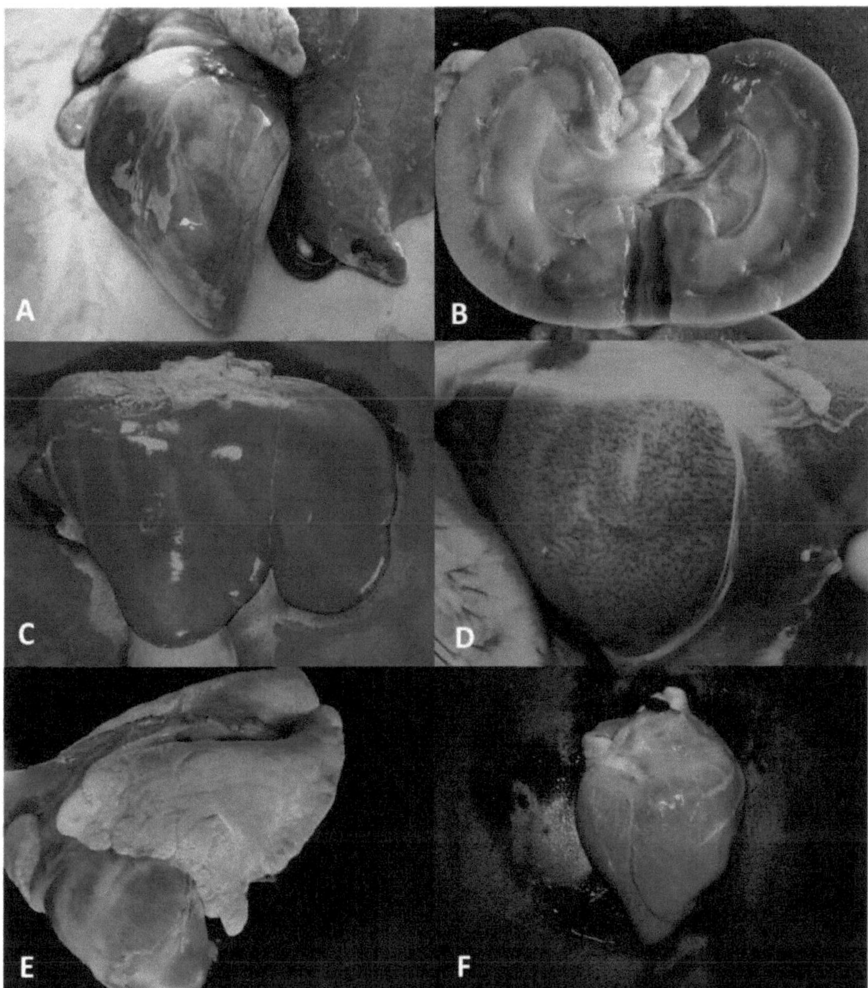

Figure 1 - Macroscopic lesions in goats chronically intoxicated by Palicourea marcgravii. A) marked multifocal to coalescent myocardial pallor. B) marked diffuse renal pallor. C) diffuse hepatic congestion. D) marked hepatic lobular pattern, E) hydropericardium. F) serous fat atrophy.

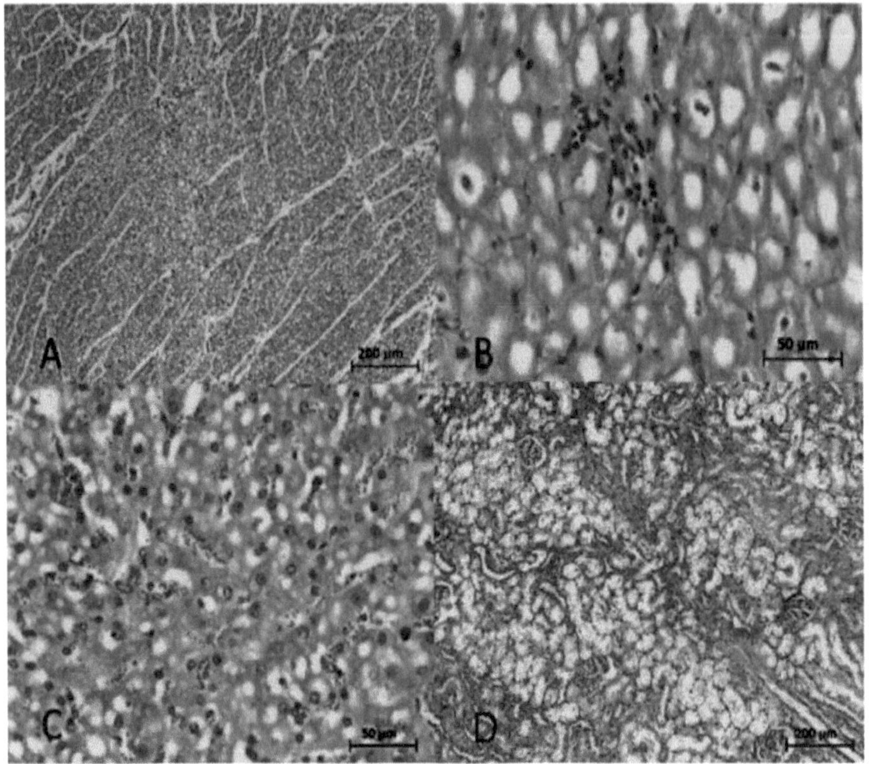

Figure 2 - Main histopathological lesions: (**A**) heart: marked multifocal to coalescent vacuolisation of cardiomyocytes, (**B**) heart: marked vacuolisation of cardiomyocytes and discrete mononuclear infiltrate, (**C**) liver: moderate vacuolar degeneration, (**D**) kidney: moderate multifocal hydropic-vacuolar degeneration of the distal convoluted tubules with karyopyknosis.

Table 1. Characteristics of intoxication and clinical signs in goats chronically intoxicated with *P. marcgravii* (Brasilia, 2013).

Animal	Sex	TDIP	Dose	ISC	CCL	Clinical signs					Outcome			
						ANX	APT	TAC	ART	TAP	VEP	PJP	DEC	
C1	M	23	4.6g/kg	19th day	5 days	+	+	+	+	+	+	+	+	E
C2	F	23	4.6g/kg	13th day	11 days	+	+	+	+	+	+	+	+	E
C3	M	38	7.6g/kg	19th day	20 days	-	-	+	+	+	+	+	+	M*
C4	M	38	7.6g/kg	23rd day	16 days	+	+	+	+	+	+	+	+	E
C5	M	38	7.6g/kg	6th day	33 days	-	+	+	+	+	+	+	+	E
C6	M	16	3.2g/k	16th	1 day	+	+	+	+	+	+	+	+	M

			g	day										
C7	M	38	7.6g/kg	26th day	13 days	+	+	+	+	+	+	+	+	M*
C8	M	30	6.0kg/kg	17th day	14 days	+	+	+	+	+	+	+	+	E
C9	M	6	1.2g/kg	5th day	2 days	-	+	+	+	+	+	-	+	M
C10	M	27	5.4g/kg	20th day	8 days	+	+	+	+	+	+	+	+	M
C11	F	-	Control	-	-	-	-	-	-	-	-	-	-	E
C12	F	-	Control	-	-	-	-	-	-	-	-	-	-	E
C13	F	-	Control	-	-	-	-	-	-	-	-	-	-	E

TDIP - total days of plant ingestion. **DTI** - total dose ingested/kg throughout the experiment. **ISC** - onset of clinical signs. CCL - duration of clinical course. * - challenge with 2g/kg. Clinical signs: **ANX** - anorexia**, APT** - apathy, **TAC** - tachycardia, **ART** - arrhythmia, **TAP** - tachypnoea, **VEP** - engorged episcleral vessels, **PJP** - positive jugular pulse**, DEC** - sternal decubitus**.** Interpretation: + present, - absent. Outcome**: M** - Died**, E** - Euthanised, **M*-** Died after challenge with 2 g/kg.

Table 2. Necroscopic changes in goats chronically intoxicated with *P. marcgravii* (Brasília, 2013).

Animal	Heart			Kidney	Liver		Lungs	
	HIP	AGG	PAM	PAL	EPL	CNG	EDM	CNG
C1	+	+	+	+	+	+	+	+
C2	+	-	+	+	+	+	+	+
C3	+	-	+	+	+	+	+	+
C4	+	-	+	+	+	+	+	-
C5	+	-	+	+	+	+	+	-
C6	+	+	+	+	+	+	+	+
C7	+	-	+	+	+	+	+	+
C8	+	-	+	+	+	+	+	-
C9	-	-	+	+	+	+	+	-
C10	+	+	+	+	+	+	-	-
C11	-	-	-	-	-	-	+	-

Clinical signs**: HIP** - hydropericardium**, AGG** - gelatinous fat atrophy, **PAM** - myocardial pallor, **PAL** - renal pallor, **EPL** - lobular pattern, **CNG** - congestion, **EDM** - oedema. Interpretation + present, - absent.

Table 3. Cardiac histopathological changes in goats chronically intoxicated with *P. marcgravii* (Brasília, 2013).

Animal	ATDR			ATEQ			SEPINT			VTDR			VTEQ		
	NIC	TVAC	INFM	NIC	TVAC	INFM	NIC	TVAC	INFM	NIC	TVAC	INFM	NIC	TVAC	INFM
C1	+	+	-	-	++	+	++	++	+	+	+	+	+	+++	+
C2	+	+	+	+	++	+	+	+++	+	+	+++	+	+	+++	+
C3	+	+	-	-	-	-	-	+	-	+	+	+	+	+	+
C4	-	+	++	-	+	+	+	+++	+	+	+++	+	+	+++	+
C5-	-	+	+	+	+	+	+	++	+	+	+++	+	+	++	+
C6	+	+	+	+	+	+	++	+++	+	++	+++	+	+	+++	+
C7	-	-	-	-	+	-	+	+	-	+	+	-	+	+	-
C8	-	-	+	-	+	+	+	+++	+	+	+	+	+	+++	+
C9	+	-	+	+	+	+	++ +	++	+	++	+	+	++	++	++
C10	+	+	-	+	+	-	++	+++	+	+	+	+	+	+++	+
C11	-	-	-	-	-	-	-	-	-	-	-	-	-	-	-

Anatomical region: **ATDR** - right atrium, **ATEQ** - left atrium, **SEPINT** - interventricular septum, **VTDR** - right ventricle, **VTEQ** - left ventricle. Histopathological changes: **CIN** - individual cardiomyocyte necrosis**, TVAC** - cardiomyocyte swelling and vacuolisation**, INFM** - mononuclear inflammatory infiltrate. Intensity: - No change**,** + slight, ++ moderate**,** +++ marked.

CHAPTER 6

DISCUSSION

This experimental model, with the ingestion of low and repeated doses of P. marcgravii, caused clinical signs, severe pathological alterations and the death of goats. It was observed that goats are also sensitive to chronic intoxication by P. marcgravii, as well as to its cumulative effect for the species, with clinical signs similar to those observed in cattle in acute intoxication (Tokarnia & Dobereiner, 1986) and sheep (Tokarnia et al. 1986). In an experiment carried out with sheep intoxicated with MFA, it did not have a cumulative effect, but the clinical and histopathological signs were similar (Shultz et al. 1982).

The daily dose of 0.2 g/kg of fresh leaves of the plant caused intoxication and clinical signs in all the animals. This dose was effective in producing the chronic form of intoxication in most of the animals, which were euthanised or died between 23 and 38 days of the experiment. Only the C6 and C9 goats died more quickly, with total amounts of plant ingested close to those considered toxic for the species and which usually lead to death within minutes to 2 days (Tokarnia et al. 1991). According to these findings, it was determined that 1.2 g/kg of fresh leaves was the minimum dose to produce death in animals after 6 days of administration. Therefore, considering that a daily dose of 0.2 g/kg of live weight of fresh leaves was administered, this corresponded to approximately 1/6 of the minimum toxic dose.

For most species, the classic form of intoxication occurs within minutes to a few hours after administration of the plant, in cattle at doses from 0.6g/kg (Tokarnia & Dobereiner, 1986), in sheep 0.5 to 1.0g/kg (Tokarnia et a. 1986), in buffalo 3.0g/kg (Barbosa et al. 2003) and in horses 0.6g/kg (Tokarnia et al. 1993). The goats in the experiment certainly developed a chronic form of P. marcgravii toxicosis, since the clinical signs appeared between 5 and 26 days after administration of the plant.

Among the clinical signs observed in chronically intoxicated goats, anorexia, apathy, tachycardia, arrhythmia, tachypnoea, positive jugular venous stasis and decubitus are alterations frequently described in ruminants naturally and experimentally intoxicated by the plant (Pacheco & Carneiro 1932, Tokarnia & Dobereiner 1986, Tokarnia et al. 1991, Barbosa et al. 2003). However, the goats showed clinical signs gradually and daily during the experiment, rather than sudden signs and nerve alterations as in the acute form (Tokarnia et al. 1991). The presence of engorged episcleral vessels is not a finding reported in the acute intoxication of goats by the plant (Tokarnia et al. 1991, Oliveira et al. 2013).

Despite the differences between the acute and chronic clinical forms of intoxication, the effects on the cardiovascular system were particularly marked and severe in the chronic form of P. marcgravii toxicosis. Unlike the acute form generally observed in ruminants, chronically intoxicated goats did not show neuromuscular alterations such as pedal movements, opisthotonus and muscle tremors (Tokarnia et al. 1991, Soto-Blanco et al. 2004, Vasconcelos et al. 2008, Peixoto et al. 2012, Becker et al. 2013).

Animals chronically intoxicated by P. marcgravii that died or were euthanised showed macroscopic lesions mainly in the heart, liver, lungs and kidneys. Of particular note are the cardiac alterations, characterised by moderate to marked pallor in the form of striations or extensive foci, which have been described sporadically in experimentally intoxicated goats (Pacheco & Carneiro 1932, Tokarnia et al. 1991).

Reproduction of acute experimental intoxication in sheep, using only MFA instead of the plant, produced venous congestion, cyanosis, pulmonary oedema, hydropericardium, hydrothorax, ascites and discrete areas of haemorrhage in the heart. In the subacute and chronic form of MFA intoxication, the myocardium can show pale spots all over the organ (Shultz et al. 1982). Some of the alterations found in the goats were similar to those found mainly in sheep intoxicated by MFA. It is important to emphasise that the cardiac pallor observed in the chronic form of P. marcgravii intoxication was similar to that described in sheep with chronic experimental MFA toxicosis (Shultz et. al. 1982).

The alterations observed in the liver and lungs of chronically intoxicated goats are possibly secondary to the lesions found to varying degrees in the myocardium. This could be demonstrated by venous congestion (clinically evidenced as stasis and jugular pulse), oedema and degeneration in the central lobular region of the liver (with evidence of a lobular pattern), the latter possibly due to hypoxia. These alterations may be observed in goats and sheep intoxicated by plants containing MFA (Tokarnia et al. 1991, Becker et al. 2013, Oliveira et al. 2013). However, these changes are not reported in the majority of cases of ruminant toxicosis caused by MFA-containing plants in Brazil, possibly because the acute or hyperacute form of poisoning predominates (Soto-Blanco et al. 2004, Peixoto et al. 2012, Becker et al. 2013, Oliveira et al. 2013).

The marked renal pallor found in the animals in the experiment is an alteration not described in ruminants intoxicated by plants containing MFA in Brazil and other parts of the world (Schultz et al. 1982, Vasconcelos et al. 2008, Peixoto et al. 2012, Oliveira et al, 2013, Duarte et al. 2014).Histopathological examination of the tissues of goats chronically intoxicated by P. marcgravii showed severe heart lesions, renal, hepatic and pulmonary alterations.

In the chronic experimental intoxication of goats with P. marcgravii leaves, the most commonly affected cardiac region was the interventricular septum, with lesions of greater intensity, followed by the left and right ventricles. The right and left atria also showed the same alterations, but with less frequency and intensity. To date, such severe lesions and their distribution in the hearts of ruminants intoxicated by MFA-containing plants have not been described in Brazil, although most studies have focused on the acute form of intoxication (Vasconcelos et al. 2008, Peixoto et al. 2012, Becker et al. 2012, Oliveira et al. 2013). So far, it is not known why there are differences in the distribution and intensity of the lesions in the cardiac areas assessed in chronically intoxicated goats. One possible explanation could be the existence of differences in the metabolic rate of cardiomyocytes or in the permeability of the membranes to the toxin in the regions assessed, which could interfere with the speed of action and distribution of the MFA (Buffa et al. 1977).

Among the histopathological changes found, tumefaction and vacuolisation of the cardiomyocytes, with multifocal to diffuse distribution and varying degrees, were the predominant lesions in 100% of the intoxicated goats. These alterations, the way they were found, have only been described previously in a similar study with goats in the Federal District (Reis jr et al. 2009). In acute experimental intoxication of goats with the plant, cardiomyocyte vacuolisation to a slight degree was reported in less than 30% of the animals (Tokarnia et al. 1991).

In the experimental intoxication of Merino sheep with sodium fluoracetate in South Africa, prominent histopathological lesions were found mainly in the endocardium, characterised by swelling of cardiac fibres, particularly in the perinuclear region, and loss of transverse striations (Schultz et al. 1982). MFA intoxication causes a marked accumulation of citrate in the tissues, caused by the blockage of the Krebs cycle, linked to the respiratory and metabolic activity of the organ, mainly in the myocardium, the nervous system, and to a lesser extent in the liver (Goncharov et al. 2006). The vacuolisation of the cardiomyocytes may have occurred due to an increase in tissue citrate, as well as the interruption of the Krebs cycle, which causes a depletion in tissue ATP levels and the accumulation of intracellular fluid.

Apparently, when examined under light microscopy, the vacuolisation seen in the goats' cardiomyocytes suggests cellular oedema. However, in an ultrastructural study of the myocardium of goats chronically intoxicated by P. marcgravii, dilation of the smooth endoplasmic reticulum was demonstrated, unlike the mitochondrial lesion usually expected (Reis jr et al. 2009).

Individual cardiomyocyte necrosis in goats chronically intoxicated by P. marcgravii was another important lesion and was similar in distribution to cardiomyocyte swelling and vacuolisation. Necrosis of cardiac fibres had previously been described in 50% of goats acutely intoxicated by the plant (Tokarnia et al. 1991). This lesion is observed in other ruminants intoxicated by plants containing MFA (Tokarnia et al. 1986, Oliveira et al. 2012), however, it is not necessarily always found (Barbosa et al. 2003, Ecco et al. 2004, Vasconcelos et al. 2008, Becker et al. 2013). Experimental intoxication of sheep with MFA also caused necrosis of cardiac fibres along the atrial and ventricular walls, most commonly affecting the endocardium. The mechanisms responsible for cell death in animals intoxicated by MFA and plants containing it occur due to the impairment of stages of cellular respiration (Colicho-Zuanaze & Satake 2005). In this situation, the death of cardiomyocytes is an expected phenomenon, due to the intense response and susceptibility of the heart to the action of MFA (Schultz et al. 1982, Goncharov et al. 2006).

The inflammatory process found in the heart of goats chronically intoxicated by the plant is also reported in the acute intoxication of these animals by P. marcgravii (Tokarnia et al. 1991), in sheep (Tokarnia et al. 1986) and in cattle (Tokarnia & Dobereiner 1986). Sheep experimentally intoxicated by MFA also showed a mononuclear inflammatory infiltrate in the myocardium (Schultz et al. 1982). The migration of inflammatory cells is possibly related to the necrosis of cardiac fibres caused by MFA.

Interstitial fibrosis in the myocardium of the animals in the experiment was a rare finding, and can be found sporadically in sheep and goats acutely intoxicated by the plant (Tokarnia et al. 1986, Tokarnia et al. 1991). Fibroplasia/fibrosis in these cases probably occurs due to the disappearance of cardiac fibres due to necrosis and replacement by fibrous tissue (Tokarnia et al. 1991).

Cattle and sheep naturally poisoned by other plants containing MFA, such as Amorimia exotropica and Amorimia sepium, show cardiomyocyte necrosis, interstitial mononuclear inflammation and severe cardiac fibrosis (Soares et al. 2011, Schons et al. 2012). This last lesion can be reproduced and exacerbated experimentally in rabbits by administering the plant for 40 days (Soares et al. 2011). Fibrosis appears in areas of necrosis and inflammation of the myocardium in sheep intoxicated chronically or subacutely by MFA, and appears sporadically in acute intoxication (Schultz et al. 1982).

It is impossible not to notice the marked differences in the predominant cardiac histological lesions in goats chronically intoxicated by P. marcgravii and ruminants intoxicated by Amorimia spp. A possible explanation for this could be the difference in the concentrations of MFA present in the two plant species. P. marcgravii has 0.21% to 0.24% MFA in its composition, much higher levels than those observed in various species of Amorimia spp. which range from 0.0007% to 0.02% (Lee et al. 2012). Even in chronic intoxications, the high concentrations of MFA in P. marcgravii, which can be 10 times or more higher than that present in Amorimia spp. probably cause the marked swelling and vacuolisation of cardiomyocytes. It is likely that lower doses of MFA induce cardiac fibrosis to an accentuated degree through mechanisms that are not yet known. If we consider the average levels of MFA in P. marcgravii (Lee et al. 2012), the dose ingested by chronically intoxicated goats was still much higher than that given to sheep, which also caused cardiac fibrosis as the main lesion (Schultz et al. 1982).

Diffuse hydropic-vacuolar degeneration (DHV) of the epithelial cells of the renal tubules was observed in a marked and constant manner in all the chronically intoxicated goats. This alteration is frequently described in ruminants intoxicated by the plant (Tokarnia et al. 1983, 1986, 1981, Tokarnia & Dobereiner, 1986, Barbosa et al. 2003, Ecco et al. 2004, Oliveira et al. 2013), in animals intoxicated with other plants containing MFA (Vasconcelos et al. 2008, Becker et al. 2013) and experimentally with the isolated use of MFA (Nogueira et al. 2010, Peixoto et al.2012).

It is important to emphasise that this lesion is usually described as focal or multifocal, affecting only the distal convoluted tubules, unlike what was observed in the goats in this experiment, which diffusely involved the tubules from the renal cortex to the cortico-medullary transition. The distribution pattern found for hydropic-vacuolar degeneration was possibly due to the prolonged administration of P. marcgravii to the goats. It is likely that chronic intoxication of the animals leads to the development of renal damage that is broader and less selective than that found in the acute form generally described in ruminants (Tokarnia et al. 1986, 1991, Tokarnia & Dobereiner 1986).

Hydropic-vacuolar degeneration was observed in all chronically intoxicated goats, but in the acute form it was found in only 36% of the animals (Tokarnia et al. 1986). Ruminants intoxicated by other toxic plants that have MFA in Brazil showed DHV ranging from 25 to 100 per cent of the animals (Tokarnia et al. 1983, 1986, 1991, Tokarnia & Dobereiner, 1986, Barbosa et al. 2003, Ecco et al. 2004, Oliveira et al. 2013). All cattle experimentally poisoned by MFA showed hydropic-vacuolar degeneration in the distal renal convoluted tubules (Nogueira et al. 2010, Peixoto et al. 2012). Differences in susceptibility, toxic dose, form of intoxication (acute or chronic) and even the plant used could explain the wide variations found in intoxicated animals.

Centrilobular vacuolisation of hepatocytes was a rare finding in chronically intoxicated goats and can be found more frequently in acute P. marcgravii intoxication in this species (Tokarnia et al. 1991). However, this lesion was not observed in sheep experimentally intoxicated by MFA (Shultz et al. 1982). Vacuolisation of hepatocytes in animals intoxicated by MFA may or may not be related to the effect of the toxin, since hypoxia associated with congestive heart failure cannot be ruled out as a cause (Nogueira et al. 2010).

Pulmonary oedema was a frequent finding in goats chronically intoxicated by P. marcgravii, and is possibly the result of damage and cardiac functional alterations caused by chronic intoxication with the plant.

Repeated administration of low doses of plants containing MFA, in order to increase the concentration of rumen bacteria producing dehalogenase, has been used successfully to prevent intoxication in ruminants (Oliveira et al. 2013, Duarte et al. 2014). However, the chronically intoxicated goats (C3 and C7) did not resist the challenge, regardless of whether or not they had undergone a detoxification period. One reason for this could be that the challenged animals received a single high dose, unlike resistance induction protocols, where the total dose was fractionated (Oliveira et al. 2013, Duarte et al. 2014). In any case, it is important to carefully administer plants containing MFA, even when used preventively, so that chronic intoxication of the animals does not occur.

The set of alterations observed in goats chronically intoxicated by P. marcgravii reflects, in an often exacerbated form, clinical manifestations and lesions known from the ingestion of plants containing MFA or the toxin itself. Low doses of the plant over a prolonged period are toxic and cause severe heart damage and death in goats. Although acute intoxication by P. marcgravii is well documented and well known, it is believed that the chronic form of intoxication can occur in field conditions, especially when the plant is in short supply or sporadically available. Even though the plant is highly palatable to ruminants, the repeated ingestion of low doses, with more discreet clinical manifestations than in the acute form of intoxication, should be considered in the differential diagnosis in the death of animals with access to forests containing P. marcgravii.

In view of the relevant findings in chronically intoxicated goats, there is an urgent need to investigate the importance of this form of intoxication in other ruminant species of greater economic importance in Brazilian livestock farming and which suffer losses from the plant. This could be extended to other plants with MFA that cause damage to various livestock regions in the country.

To the National Research Council (CNPq) for financial support. Project funded by the Institute of Science and Technology for the Control of Plant Poisoning (Proc. CNPq 573534/2008-0).

CHAPTER 7

REFERENCES

Alzert, S.P., A review of sodium monoflouracetate its properties, toxicology and use on predator and control. Special scientific Report on Wildlife 146. U.S. Department of the Interior, 1971

Barbosa, R. R.; Ribeiro Filho, M. R.; Da Silva, I. P.; Soto-Blanco, B. Toxic plants of interest to livestock: Importance and ways of studying them. Acta Veterinária Brasílica, v.1, n.1, p.1-7, 2007.

Barbosa, J. D., Oliveira, C.M.C., Tokarnia H. C., 2003. Comparison of the sensitivity of cattle and buffalo to intoxication by Palicourea marcgravii (Rubiaceae) Pesquisa Veterinária Brasileira, Seropédical, v.23, n.4, 167-172.

Becker, M., Caldeira F.H.B., Carneiro, F.M., Oliveira, L.P., Tokarnia C.H., Riet-Correa F., Lee, S.T & Colodel, E.M. 2013. Importance of Amorimia publfora (Malpighiaceae) intoxication in cattle in Mato GrossoSul: experimental reproduction of intoxication in sheep and cattle. Pesquisa Veterinária Brasileira, v.33, n9, p.1049-1056.

Buffa, P. Pasquali-Ronchetti I. Biochemical Lesions of Respiratory Enzymes and Configurational Changes of Mitochondrial in vivo. Cell Tissue Res., v.183, p. 1-23, 1977.

Collichio-Zuanaze R.C. Satake M. Clinical and therapeutic aspects of sodium fluoroacetate intoxication in domestic animals: Review. Vet. Not. v. 11, n.2 p.81-89, 2005

Camboim, E. K. a, Almeida, A. P., Tadra-Sfeir, M. Z., Junior, F. G., Andrade, P. P., McSweeney, C. S., ... Riet-Correa, F. (2012). Isolation and identification of sodium fluoroacetate degrading bacteria from caprine rumen in Brazil. TheScientificWorldJournal, 2012, 178254. doi:10.1100/2012/178254

Camboim E.K.A., Tadra-Sfeir M.Z., Souza E.M., Pedrosa F.O., Andrade P. P., McSweeney C.S.,

Riet-Corea F. & Melo M.A. 2012a. Defluorination of sodium fluoroacetate by bacteria from soil and plants in Brazil. Scientific World Journal. Article ID 149893, 5 pages, Available at <http://www.tswj.com/2012/149893/> Accessed 20 Aug. 2012. doi:10.1100/2012/149893

Chenoweth M.B.; Monofluoracetic acid and related compounds . Pharmacological Reviews, v.1 p383-424, 1949.

National Council for the Control of Animal Experimentation - CONCEA. Ministry of Science, Technology and Innovation. CONCEA Euthanasia Practice Guidelines. Brasilia, 2013.

Duarte A.L. L., Medeiros R.M.T., Carvalho F.K.L., Lee S. T., Cook D., Pfister J.A., Costa V.M.M., Riet-Corrêa F. Induction and transfer of resistance to poisoning by Amorimia (Mascagnia) septentrionalis in goats. Journal Applied Toxicology. 2014 Feb;34(2):220-3. doi: 10.1002/jat.2860. Epub 2013 Feb 12.

Ecco R., Túry E., Santos M.M. & Barros R.M. 2004. Palicourea marcgravii intoxication in cattle associated with cerebral malacia. Pesquisa Veterinária Brasileira. v.24 p.20-21.

Eason C.T., Gooneratne R., Fitzgerald H., Wright G., Frampton C. 1994. Persistence of sodium monofluoracetate in livestock animals and risk to humans. Human & Experimental Toxicology . 13:119-122.

Egyed M.N. & Schutlz R.A. 1986. The efficacy of acetamide for treatment of experimental Dichapetalum cymosum (Giblaar) poisoning in sheep. Onderstepoort Journal of Veterinary Research. 53:231-234.

Goncharov, N. V., Jenkins, R.O., Radilov, A. S. Toxicology of fluoracetate: review, with possible directions for therapy research.JornalOf Applied Toxocology, v 26: 148-161, 2006.

Gooneratne S.R., Eason C.T., Dickson C.J., Fitzgerald H., Wright G. 1995. Persistence of sodium monoflouracetate in rabbits and risk to non-target species. Human & Experimental Toxicology. 14: 212-216.

Kemmerling, W. Toxicity of Palicourea marcgravii: combined effects of fluoroacetate, N-methyltyramine and 2-methyltetrahydro-beta-carboline. Zeitschrift fur Naturforschung, v. 51, p. 59-64, 1996.

Kellerman,T.S.; Coetzer, J.A.W.; Naude,T.W.; Botha, C.J. Plant Poisonings and mycotoxicoses of livestock in Southern Africa. 2nd ed. Oxford University Press, Cape Town. 2005.

Krebs H.C., Kemmerling W. & Habermehl G. 1994. Qualitative and quantitative determination of fluoroacetic acid in Arrabidea bilabiata and Palicourea marcgravii by F-NMR spectroscopy. Toxicon 32: 909-913.

Lee S.T., Cook D., Riet-Correa F., Pfister J.A., Anderson W.R., Lima F.G. & Gardner 8 D. 2012. Detection of monofluoracetate in Palicourea and Amorimia species. 9 Toxicon 60:791-796.

Minnaar P.P. Swan G.E., McCrindle R.I , de Beer W.H.J. , Naudé T.W. , A High-Performance Liquid Chromatographic Method for the Determination of Monofluoroacetate. Journal of Chromatographic Science, Vol. 38, January 2000.

Nogueira V.A., França T.N., Peixoto T. C., Caldas S.A., Armién A.G. & Peixoto P.V. 2010. Experimental intoxication by sodium monofluoroacetate in cattle: clinical and pathological aspects. Pesquisa Veterinária Brasileira. v.30(7)p.533-540.

Oliveira M.M. 1963. Chromatographic isolation of monofluoroacetic acid from Palicourea marcgravii, St. Hill. Experientia 19(11):586-587.

Oliveira C. M. C. De Barbosa, J. D., Macedo R. S. C., Brito M. F.B., Peixoto P.V., & Tokarnia C.H. (2004). Comparative study of the toxicity of Palicourea juruana (Rubiaceae) to buffalo and cattle, Pesquisa Veterinária Brasileira. v. 24(1)p. 27-30.

Oliveira M.D., Riet-Correa, F. Carvalho, F.K., Silva G.B., Pereira W.S., Medeiros R.M.T. 2013. Induction of resistance to intoxication by Palicourea aeneosfusca (Rubiaceae) through administration of successive non-toxic doses. Pesquisa Veterinária Brasileira. v.33(6)p.731-

734.

Pacheco G. & Carneiro V.1932. Experimental studies on toxins. I Intoxication of animals by "erva de rato da mata" Revista Soc. Paulista de Medicina Veterinária. 2(2/3):23-46.

Pattison F.L.M. 1959 Toxic Aliphatic fluoride compouds. Elsevier: London.

Peixoto, T. C., Oliveira, L. I., Caldas, S. A., Catunda, F. E. A., Carvalho, M. G., & França, T. N. 2011. Protective effect of acetamide on experimental poisoning in rats by sodium monofluoroacetate and by some Brazilian plants that cause sudden death. Pesquisa Veterinária Brasileira. 31(11), 938-952.

Peixoto, T.C.; Nogueira, V.A.; Caldas, S.A.; França, T.N.; Anjos, B.L.; Aragão, A.P.; Peixoto, P.V. 2012. Protective effect of acetamide in cattle indicates monofluoracetate as toxic principle of Palicourea marcgravii (Rubiaceae). Pesquisa Veterinária Brasileira. April 2012 V.32(4), p.319-328.

Peixoto, T. C.; Oliveira M. L. I.; Caldas, S. A.; Catunda Jr, F. E. A.; Mario G. Carvalho, T. N. F. E. P. V.P.; Carvalho, J. M. G.; França, T. N.; Peixoto, P. V. Protective effect of acetamide on experimental intoxications in rats by sodium monoluoroacetate and by some Brazilian plants that cause sudden death. Pesquisa Veterinária Brasileira. Rio de Janeiro, v. 31, n. 11, p. 15, 2011.

Passos D.A. 1983. Experimental poisoning in goats (Capra hircus) by Palicoure aeneofusca (M.Arg.) Standl. (Rubiaceae). Master's thesis, Univ. Fed. Rural de Pernambuco, Recife, PE. 40p.

Riet-Correa F. & Medeiros R.M.T. 2001. Plant poisoning in ruminants in Brazil and Uruguay: economic importance, control and risks to public health. Pesquisa Veterinária Brasileira. v.21,p.38-42.

Pessoa C.R.M., Medeiros R.M.T., Riet-Correa F. Economic importance, epidemiology and control of plant poisoning in Brazil. Pesquisa Veterinária Brasileira. 33(6):752-758, June 2013, v. 33,

p. 752-758.

Reis Jr.J.L., Castro M.B., Moscardini A.C., Novais E.P.F., Borges J.R.J., Riet-Correa F., Howerth E. W. Histopathologic and Ultrastructural Findings of chronic experimental Cardiotoxicity Induced By Monofluoracetate Producing-Plant Palicourea marcravii. AAAVLD Annual Conference Proceedings 52 ed. 2009. p.169.

Schons S.V., Lopes T.V., Melo T.L., Lima J.P., Riet-Correa F., Barros M.A.B., Schild A.L.P. Plant poisoning in ruminants and horses in the central region of Rondônia. Ciencia Rural. V.42, n.7, p.1257-1263, jul, 2012

Soares M.P., Pavarini S.P.,Adrien M.L., Quevedo P.S., Schild A.L., Peixoto P.V., Cruz C.E.F., Driemeier D. Amorimia exotropica poisoning as a presumptive cause of myocardial fibrosis in cattle. J.VET.Diagn. Invest. 2011 23: 1226. DOI:10.1177 1040638711425586.

Soifer A.l., Kostyniak P.J. 1983. The enzymatic defluorination of fluoracetate in mouse liver cytosol: the separation of defluorination activity from several glutathione S-transferases of mouse liver. Archives of Biochemistry and Biophysics.v. 225, p.928-953.

Soto-Blanco B., Haraguchi M., Silva J.A., Gorniak L. S. Natural intoxication of goats and sheep by P. marcgravii (Rubiaceae). Revista Caatinga. 2004; 17(1):52-56.

Shultz, R. A., Coetzer, W. Kellerman, Y.S., Naudé, T.W. Observations on the clinical, cardiac and histopathological effects in sheep. Onderstepoort Journal of Veterinay Research, 49, 237-245, 1982.

Tokarnia, C. H.; Dobereiner, J.; Couceiro J.E.M. & Silva A.C.C. 1983. Intoxication by *Palicourea aeneofusca* (Rubiaceae) the cause of " sudden deaths in cattle in the Zona da Mata of Pernambuco. Pesquisa Veterinária Brasileira. 3(3): 75-79.

Tokarnia, C.H., Peixoto, P.V., Dobereiner, J. Experimental intoxication by *Palicourea marcgravii* (Rubiaceae) in sheep. Pesquisa Veterinária Brasileira, v. 6, p. 121-131, 1986.

Tokarnia, C.H., Peixoto, P.V. & Dobereiner, J. Plantas que afetam o funcionamento do coração de bovinos no Brasil. Pesquisa Veterinária Brasileira. v.10, p. 1-10, 1990.

Tokarnia, C.H., Peixoto, P.V., Dobereiner, J. Experimental intoxication by *Palicourea marcgravii* (Rubiaceae) in goats. Pesquisa Veterinária Brasileira, v. 11, p. 65-70, 1991.

Tokarnia C.H., Costa E.R., Barbosa J.D., Armien A.G.,& Peixoto P.V. 1993. Experimental poisoning by *Palicourea marcgravii* (Rubiaceae) in horses. Pesq. Vet. Bras. 13: 67-72.

Tokarnia C.H., Brito, M.F. Barbosa, J.D. Peixoto P.V. Dobereiner J., Plants that affect heart function. In. Toxic Plants of Brazil. 1. ed. Rio de Janeiro: Helianthus, 2012. p.27-37.

Vasconcelos J.S., Riet-Correa F., Dantas A.F., Medeiros R.M.T. & Dantas A.J.A. 2008. 34 Sudden deaths in cattle caused by Palicourea aeneofusca (Rubiaceae) and Mascagnia rígida (Malpighiaceae) in the Zona da Mata Paraibana. Pesquisa Veterinária Brasileira. 28, 457-460.

Vickery B, Vickery M.L. Fluoride metabolism in Dichapetalum toxicarium. Phytochemitry. 1972, v.11, p.1905-1909.

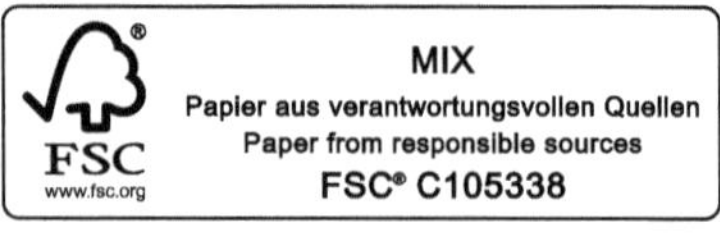

Printed by Books on Demand GmbH, Norderstedt / Germany